Guide to
Muscular Healing

Theresa L. Brumfield

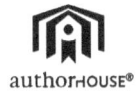

authorHOUSE®

AuthorHouse™
1663 Liberty Drive
Bloomington, IN 47403
www.authorhouse.com
Phone: 1-800-839-8640

First published by AuthorHouse 6/18/2010

ISBN: 978-1-4520-2769-2 (e)
ISBN: 978-1-4520-2770-8 (sc)

Library of Congress Control Number: 2010907878

Printed in the United States of America
Bloomington, Indiana

This book is printed on acid-free paper.

I'm sincerely grateful to 2 individuals.

Anthony Motley for spending 2 years working his massage magic and getting me out of daily pain.

Michael Clausen for giving me hope that healing was possible and referring to my problems as structural which was the key to healing.

Table of Contents

Author's Note

THIS GUIDE IS DESIGNED TO assist you in your muscular healing process. Each of us has our own past injuries that have shaped us. I wanted to write this in a way that it could help someone with long-term pain as well as someone who feels that they need to know what to look for and practice prevention and maintenance.

Obviously, everyone feels changes as they age, and this guide can aid you to aging gracefully.

I also mentioned the medical profession because getting help is always best. But I found that doctors really don't want to deal with these issues and just advise rest and pain medication. There were times where I felt the medical people treated you as if you were making it all up or it was just in your head. As if they didn't want to believe that someone could have chronic pain that was really just that chronic pain.

My personal struggles with my long-term pain are touched on in this guide as an example. And it has been my determination to heal that brings awareness to certain factors that can help anyone at any stage in their healing. My sincere hope is that the people who read this can heal as well. Be determined and be in charge.

Do You Have Chronic Muscle Pain???

DOCTORS WOULD TELL YOU TO take anti-inflammatory and aspirin. But I'm not a doctor, I'm a regular person like you that has had chronic muscle pain and beat it. You ask: How did I beat it? I beat it by taking my health into my own hands. By being in charge enough to figure out how to fix my pain.

I had a severe problem with my neck. It reached a climax when my right arm stopped working and was like a dead noodle. I tried cortisone shot in the neck, I tried chiropractic, I tried acupuncture, and I tried massage. I would say that each had an effect except the shot in the neck, but in the end it was my persistence and ingenuity that allowed me to heal.

Let me explain why. I discovered that the body as a mechanism is constantly trying to find balance between its right and left side. When you injure one side, it literally impacts both sides because change occurs to find a new balance. Muscles kick in to cover for the injured part, more muscle is created to find balance. My personal experience was that I literally had one bad muscle on top of one another, layers upon layers trying to do one thing, find balance. Now my condition was so bad the masseuses gave up working on my neck and my doctor compared it to piano wire, so in my case the acupuncture was necessary to allow the masseuse to make a change to the muscle.

I know there are a lot of techniques to changing muscle, to get it to release or relax. However, the one technique that really works is to apply steady pressure to the knotted area and just wait it out until it caves or releases. My masseuse actually spent 90 minutes holding on one muscle with his elbow to get it to loosen up, it was just that locked up. And when you are in really bad shape each release does take awhile, however the release you'll feel is like a breath of fresh air. And you can assist in the process by taking big deep breaths and staying calm.

In my case I needed 4 years of massage and at times I couldn't afford the masseuse. When that happens, use a knobble, it's a muscle tool that allows you to place the rounded point to the problem muscle and use the floor as the wedge. Any immovable surface can act as the wedge. You have to find what works for you. As long as the muscle is trapped and has constant pressure, the muscle will release. So yes, you can do this alone, with no cost to you besides buying the $10.00 muscle tool. I know some people aren't comfortable with paying for massage and that's OK as long as you have a way to take care of yourself and this is how you do it.

The days of popping a pill for temporary relief need to go. The body gives us pain to tell us something is wrong and it is up to us to listen and respond. By covering up the pain with a pill we never resolve the problem. We need to start caring for the body in finding the imbalance. And usually there are 3 points affected by a problem spot. Where the pain is coming from is one, then there are to 2 spots on the opposite side. All 3 spots need work because they are acting as a team. And often when the knobble is in location, the 2 other spots can flare up to tell you where they are, and it is handy to have more than one knobble so that you can work the body's balance system by releasing both sides of your body, because one bad muscle on one side has a best friend helping him out on the other side. And you'll find thru experimentation, that when you have 2 muscles trapped, a third muscle (a close neighbor) will kick in that wasn't participating before because it's trying to pick up the slack of what the trapped muscle can't do. The body's natural tendency is always to activate a muscle when the body is out of balance or another muscle needs assistance. This can create overlapping bad muscles. Just as the body can create bone where there is deficiencies, the body can also create more muscle. Whereas ideally, we want the original muscle relaxed and working properly then to have one bad tissue over another. My neck was huge with bad muscle and once corrected, my neck became half the size. People thought I had lost weight and all that happened was my neck shrunk.

Even after doing all the muscle work, I found there were still imbalances. I used a weighted tubular bar and placed it in different locations and found more locked up muscles, muscles that I never thought would be impacted by the neck, such as having bad muscles under and to the left of the sternum. The weighted bar allowed those muscles to relax, muscles that I didn't even know existed. So, in essence, it takes some experimentation with your body to find all of the imbalances. And sometimes they aren't even near each other.

Every one of my past injuries played a part in my chronic pain, my body had distorted itself and became unbalanced. After all, pain is the body's only way of communicating with you that there is a problem. And I would say, the biggest problem out there is that we mask our pain with drugs instead of searching for and correcting the muscular problem that caused our pain to begin with.

My Theory

I HAVE THE THEORY THAT there is a way to stave off the aging process where it relates to movement and taken further can prevent osteoporosis. And I don't mean by the act of exercise. I mean by making changes to the body to give it better alignment and balance and correcting structural problems. Chiropractors have tried to use this approach, but have failed in the attempt, their result is usually temporary. Masseuses have also tried this approach and failed, although they are closer. What if neither is necessary, what if what we have to fight is the body's own natural tendencies or the way it operates.

When we are born, it is called the fetus position. And as we go through life we get bigger, expand in width and height. When we reach full maturity it is said that we are in our prime and are strong and healthy, and from there, the body is on the decline, aging, slowly dying some would say. And the body responds and loses range of motion and we no longer attempt the feats of our youth.

Only temporarily off topic, I did gymnastics in my youth. I did this skill on the even bars called a Flying Hip Circle. I accidently lost control and awareness; I flew through the air and found I took on the fetal position for my crash landing. In reality all was OK, I did a Hecht over the low bar and landed on my hands and knees. I became very aware that the fetal position is the body's natural way of dealing, of protecting itself, more innate than learned.

So if that's the case, then what does the body do in aging? I submit that the body's natural way is to return to the fetal position. Older people begin to slouch, the body literally caves inward as part of the aging process. What if you could make the body return from its inward tendencies to an outstretched position? I have done this, and I have renewed movement, I have found that the parts of the body work again and with more efficiency. I feel younger, while at the same time, I also feel the body does still age, but with less of a price.

I then contemplated osteoporosis. I believe that because the body caves inward with age and injury, it is creating a change to the bones. Through my chiropractic experience, I have found that the muscles are usually to blame for the sublexations that occur. Through either injury or aging, the muscles become out of balance and put pressures on the bones to make adjustments. Where chiropractic is successful is putting the bones back in proper alignment, however, if you don't fix the muscles first, it literally becomes useless. It seems that the muscles have the real power and can overtake the bones, which is where osteoporosis comes in. So once you put the body's tendency of moving inward into play, and muscles overtaking the bones, there is no stopping the bones from forming whatever position the muscles take them in. And this caving in is where the muscles will take them based on the body's natural tendency.

So then you ask, how did I return my body from its caving inward position? I tried something very unusual. I laid on my back on the floor, and applied a tubular weight to positions on my front that would elongate my width, to reverse the caving inward position. Using weights is a similar approach as massage, only there is no need for movement or work by a masseuse. The body's natural tendency with massage is that the pressure causes the muscle to relax. The same works with weight. Only weight is actually more effective. Sometimes it's hard to relax when someone's digging in your muscles. But with a weighted object, you are in control, and you are able to relax and the muscle works that much faster at relaxing and elongating. All you have to focus on is your breathing, nice long deep breaths. Not to mention, that a masseuse can only work one muscle at a time, whereas the weighted object can literally relax all of the muscles in its path.

Another thing I became aware of, was what I learned about bone density. I took a bone density test at 40. They kept saying the test must be reading wrong after getting the same result 4 times. They said if they read the test results as is, my bones are equivalent to a 20 yr old. Apparently the test is based on a 26 yr old and I tested far below that. Because I did gymnastics and did a lot of repetition with landings, I have to assume that old saying "Use it or Lose it" applies here. Your bones must be used to stay healthy and strong. If you are a long-term couch potato, then yes your bones are likely to deteriorate from lack of use. Simple activities such as walking are instrumental to your bone health if you are not the athletic type. For upper body bone health, you can hold the standard push-up position, doing the actual push-up is not necessary, just hold the starting position for 30 seconds and you've worked and applied weight on those upper body bones.

So in conclusion, there is ways to promote a holistic approach to gaining your movement back from its aged condition or injured condition. And I'm always in favor of exercise to promote a healthy body. But sometimes that just isn't enough, as I am proof that a life of sports is not enough. I believe in good movement for all regardless of age, so keep fighting the good fight.

The Mighty Most Overlooked Muscle

THE MUSCLE I AM REFERRING to is called the sternocleidomastoid muscle. This muscle can do a lot of damage when it is stressed and has years of neglect. I call it the most overlooked muscle because I've received massages for years and most massage therapists are afraid to work on the neck in general and when they do work the neck it's usually only the back side that they work on. Most of them will say the problem is elsewhere. When you try to pin a masseuse to working on the neck, a lot of them will tell you they don't work on the front side because there is too much health risks involved, which clearly makes this muscle ignored since it is located in the front and side of the neck. You can feel it start under the jaw out wide and travels sideways toward the throat. This muscle is a large muscle that greatly affects the smaller neighboring muscles that are finger like parts that literally grip both your front and back side almost like a claw that clamps both sides and gives you front to back stability.

It has taken me 5 years of working with an acupuncturist (electrical system) and a chiropractor (bones) and a masseuse (muscles) to overcome a long-term neck injury I sustained from gymnastics 25 years ago combined with the stresses on our neck from daily living. Each muscle in my neck needed muscle releasing and the sternocleidomastoid muscle was the most profound. I have struggled with other injuries as a result of having neck issues. As my neck has improved I have seen a huge improvement in my power game as a tennis player, but I had no idea that this muscle was threatening in other areas.

The day I had my masseuse focus on this muscle and it took over an hour to get any kind of release and I instantly smelled the candle burning in the corner of the room. The candles were always there and I have never smelled them before, considering that they were there just to provide light. I asked my masseuse if he smelled any change and said no. I feel like I have a new sense of smell now, which I certainly did not suspect. Then I noticed my jaw cracked a few times and it released and became more relaxed. 24 hours after my massage I went and played tennis, which is probably a no-no, but that's me. I have for years struggled with hot feet, and even looked for tennis shoes to promote "cool feet" and found that they did not help this problem, however, on this particular night I played as rigorous as I could and I did not experience hot feet. I had noticed tingling in my feet while getting the massage and masseuse said that's blood getting to your feet it's not use to. Then I noticed my arms didn't hurt as much as usual, however, they hurt a lot while the masseuse was working his magic. And that wasn't the end of the magic. I then woke up the next morning and something was different. My breathing. It was light, it was easy, it was deep, it was full and perfect. I had no idea that my breathing had changed, but it felt so good I just wanted to breathe all day. Now that's what I call enjoying each moment. So I ask you, how can this muscle have all this power? It also amazes me that our bodies are constantly changing with us not even noticing the changes. I had no idea that my breathing had changed over the years, it was literally like a cat lying on your chest while you slept and then the cut jumped off. The effort to breath was gone; however, you didn't realize you were having to make this effort.

So I say, please don't ignore your sternocleidomastoid muscle. Make your masseuse work on that part of your neck if that's what it needs. We all know that shoulder and neck muscles easily get fatigued while working a job. Each and every one of us could have a stressed sternocleidomastoid muscle and not even realize it. Each of us knows that the body is constantly changing as we get older and it usually is not for the better. Let's not help our body's age by ignoring the stuff we still have control over.

Why is Back Pain So Prominent

I MENTIONED EARLIER THAT THE body's natural tendency is to cave inward toward the fetal position as its innate way of dealing with injuries. I also mentioned that this caving inward is caused by the muscles and the bones alignment is affected. The caving inward is most notable with the right vs. left side of our body. But the caving inward goes further than that. It caves from top to bottom as well; from neck to pelvic region. As one's body pulls inward in this way, by creating problems with the frontal muscles and in fact shortening them; the back is left to suffer the consequences. In fact it is the frontal side that we need to care for; however, the pain we're experiencing is in the back. The back muscles are stretched, and after so long the stretched muscles feel fatigue and cause pain. While the front has no pain but form knots that cause it to be locked up and they need to be worked out. And usually the locked up frontal muscles are not budging when the back is in pain as they've had longer to cement themselves.

This brings me to another one of those powerful muscles of the body. Located just off to each side of the sternum, you will find Triangularis Sterni. The muscle runs multi-directional; at its highest portion it runs vertical, at its mid portion it runs diagonal towards the shoulder and at its lowest portion runs horizontal. I believe it's these multi-directional muscles that cause the most problems for us. The sternocleidomastoid and its smaller neighboring muscles together create multi-directional muscle strands that also causes problems.

While working on frontal muscles, flip the knobble upside down so that the wider base is against the body as you do not want the pointy end being used because things are just a little bit more delicate in the front than they are on your back side. In fact, where the frontal muscles are concerned, it is best to use the weighted tubular bar so as not to damage ribs or small muscle structures.

So essentially both these muscles pull the body in both a caving inward from top to bottom as well as caving inward from side to side. It is my belief that when one of these muscles is stressed, so is the other. And working in the same manner, can really alter your form and put a lot of stress not only on the back muscles but also on your spinal alignment especially in my case, where the issues were more one sided. My caving inward process was extreme on my left side and almost non-existent on the right side. That's why your injuries over time really have an effect on your body even when you thought it healed just fine. So my point is, you have an injury, you then heal from that injury, however, you've never addressed those changes the body made in dealing with that injury. Therefore causing the caving inward process and giving you back pain as a result because the back is the last part to be effected. You didn't feel pain in any of these other changes, because the body could adjust itself, whereas the back can't adjust itself, because to do so it would need the front to be unlocked. So think of the muscle that can't help itself as the one that cries the loudest and is usually last at trying to cement itself.

So if a large percentage of our population is experiencing back pain, it was probably because they didn't live a non-injured life. Injuries happen; I've actually never met anyone who's never had an injury. Injury is the price we pay in leading an active lifestyle. I mean if you can twist an ankle in walking off a curb, then it's pretty difficult to live a non-injured lifestyle. So it does make sense that back pain is prominent. It is only until we practice prevention and work to keep our bodies from pulling inward over time as in a life-style choice to look for signs and work at maintaining a proper posture; a poster you likely had when you were in your prime.

Are we Recognizing the Signs?

I DON'T THINK WE ARE recognizing the signs. We are so quick to take an aspirin or Advil that we don't stop and think about where this pain we are having is coming from. I was casually talking to my neighbor, telling her I was trying to heal from a long-term injury and mentioned that I was trying to get my left shoulder lower, and she mentioned she had a high shoulder too. I instantly asked her what she was doing to correct it and she said nothing and the conversation soon ended. But it got me thinking that millions of people probably have the sign of a high shoulder and think nothing of it. Well my high shoulder first caused back pain. It then caused me to have plantar fasciitis, and when I got that to heal, it then caused a hamstring injury. The body was simply passing on this weakness caused by the high shoulder to whatever territory I was giving the least amount of care to. Between my left foot and left shoulder there was too much stress. I later realized that it was my neck injury that caused the neck/shoulder union shrinking causing the high shoulder. Now we all know that the neck can be easily fatigued by the stresses of life to any average person. But does the average person get regular massages? The fact is that they don't. Most people getting massages do some sort of physical activity. And yes, by doing physical stuff, the body will react more loudly then if we are more sedentary beings. But because the body is constantly changing, to completely ignore a problem, is to allow it to get worse. I've had my high shoulder for probably 20 years and I know I wasn't born with a high shoulder. Why did I and so many others think a high shoulder is not a problem? Did we think it's a natural part of aging? Well I've had pain for 20 years, but I never connected that the pain I was experiencing was because of a high shoulder that I could physically see in the mirror. Also, by having pain that started in my back, I wanted to give care to my back and because I never found the root cause (my neck), I was allowing further degeneration.

Do we purposely ignore signs because we don't know how to fix them and as long as there's no pain, everything is OK? Do we give up on an activity because we only experience pain when doing the activity and chalk it up as aging? Is pain the deciding factor that, OK I need to do something?

Pain is always are biggest indicator of a problem. And we've learned to take an aspirin and get rest. We go to bed and feel better in the morning. Why, because the muscle is in a horizontal position and is at rest. But have you noticed that you will go to work, and whether sitting or standing all day, that by 2:00pm you start to ache again. The same muscle that was not taken care of properly, activates pain again, because it is no longer at rest, and tires again because of that deficiency you have yet to discover. If you never do anything about your pain, your body does its own form of change, pulling itself inward, causing other areas to be disturbed. And the longer you fail to deal with it, the more damage occurs in the long run. The body will always change to correct its deficiency if you ignore it, and later in life, you will find that you can no longer do the activities you once enjoyed. It seems to me that the more stuff you ignore, the more aged your body becomes. You are in charge of how it ages. Does it age gracefully or does it age with suffering and immobility.

There are many ways to watch for signs. Everybody is different and could have a different set of signs. Besides my high shoulder and not finding the root cause of my pain, there were other signs. Stand natural and comfortably in front of a mirror, look for signs. The Egoscue Center where I was measured, showed me that my feet did not have the normal stance (feet pointing forward in the same direction and less wider than shoulder width), mine were one pointing straight and other off at an angle and they were too wide apart. A wide foot stance is a sign. My arms did not equally hang on the sides of my body. We all find standing in front of a mirror for a period of time to be uncomfortable, but it is necessary when pain materializes. Use the mirror as a tool to help you discover what you can't feel on your own.

You can also lay on your back on a hard surface. When in this position, do you feel balanced from left side to right side? Do your shoulder blades touch the floor feeling the same? Do your hips feel the same? How about the part of the arm that's touching the floor, is it the same on both sides? When you lay there completely relaxed, do your feet relax in the same manner?

For any part of you that is off from one side of you to the other, see it as a sign that there is a muscular problem that needs fixing, and you'll be that closer to determining how to fix your muscular pain.

Well, I'll admit that I didn't know how to fix my pain for many years. I went on ignoring the signs on purpose as so many people do. I kept getting the occasional massage and really didn't dive in to fix my problem until my right arm completely stopped working in its normal manner.

I don't think our society has really taken on prevention as strongly as it pretends to do. We pay attention to those areas that scream the loudest. And is it easier to give your car maintenance than your own body? Please, take a moment, and consider the condition of your own body. If your body feels 10 years younger than your actual age, well, then you are in the one percentile and should consider yourself lucky, because the rest of us do not.

I hate to say this, but is it because we are overwhelmed because if the doctors can't figure everything out about the body, how can we? I can't fix my pain because I just don't know how? Well I hope I can help in this area, but I clearly understand the perspective of being overwhelmed.

Please remember that you only have one body and quite frankly, I don't think the average person learns enough about the body. So my advice is, to stop ignoring the signs, and give your body the attention it deserves.

Muscular Aging

WE ALL KNOW OUR MUSCLES change in aging. At 40 we remember that we can't run like we did at 30, and at 50 we remember we can't run like we did at 40. There are 2 questions that come to mind and one is why, what changes, and secondly can it be reversed?

My belief is that once we past our prime, our body makes negative adjustments to offset imbalances. That right handed people often have left legged tightness in the thigh and hip. By the body creating knots in the left hip, it eases the stress our dominant hand is creating. However, once the left hip engages in forming knots, other knots begin to form in other areas of the body to deal with that new change and on and on it goes, that battle our body's go through that creates muscular aging. Other things happen as well such as stress that creates a shortening of the neck/shoulder union. The neck/shoulder union creates further changes. By elongating the muscles in the neck and shoulder, you can once again have greater range of motion in the hip. So the hip changes and neck changes combat each other creating the caving inward process that people see later in life. The problem is that the caving inward process is so gradual that it can't be noticed and everyone over the age of 40 should have physical changes that are simply muscular aging, the process of the body forming knots. Injuries further the process and some injuries can send the body spiraling into chronic pain, because the body is aging irregularly or incorrectly, forming knots right and left because it can't find the balance it needs.

My situation is that through injuries my body was aging incorrectly. So I needed to reverse the bad muscle (removing all of the knots) and try to bring the body back to the correct structure, a structure that is balanced with shoulders down and wide and hips free of knots. It can be done, but it isn't an easy process. I would wish everyone to monitor those areas of the body that create the most imbalances. Also try not to be so one-sided dominant, when lifting try to center the weight so each hand has an equal share. If we as a society could reverse our knots at 40, we could continue to run like we did at 30, and the same goes for 50 and so forth. That if we could practice better prevention in the areas of our musculature our bodies would function more properly.

By allowing our body's to form extensive knot systems, we are allowing it to break down in so many ways. My losses were endless, to name a few, I experienced loss of range of motion, had chronic pain, my hair thinned, my sexuality was non-existent, my breathing was labored, my lack of smell and so on. However, all of those items listed were reversed by removing the knot systems and bringing the body back in balance and giving it the correct structure.

A funny thing I noticed was that I only needed to shave my legs once every 2-3 months while my left side was collapsed, however, once I was healed my hair growth rebounded and required me to shave my legs every 2-3 days. A pretty big difference and a great tell all for women who aren't sure of the condition they are in.

I once learned that a muscle in the eye that changes your focus from close to far and vice versa, begins to tire at the age of 45. Through muscle work you can stave off that aging function by keeping the muscle practicing, however once you stop working it, it finally succumbs to weakening and that sharp focus is more elusive. I believe our muscular body's are similar in that they work as well as we practice them to work. A process of removing knots as they come will allow us to move like we did when we were 30, however, if we fail to practice our muscles they will succumb to weakening. I believe it is our choice in how our muscular body's age.

Advantages/Disadvantages to Your Muscle Tools

YOUR 3 MUSCLE TOOLS CONSIST of the knobble, your masseuse, and a weighted tubular bar. Each has its advantages and disadvantages.

Your masseuse is a great tool when you are not sure what your trouble spots are. Ask for a full body massage and ask him/her to tell you where your knotted spots are. Many masseuses skip over a lot of areas and be sure to ask him/her to check everything, even such things as stomach muscles, front and side neck muscles, the lats, and even pectoral muscles. The key here is to be thorough. Most massages are only an hour so you don't want to waste the time having them spend a half hour on one muscle, when you can go home and use the knobble more effectively.

The reason that the knobble is more effective is because once you properly trap a muscle, it cannot wiggle free, as this happens a lot on the massage table. It is customary for a muscle to fight the process and wiggle right out of the grasp of your masseuse and this can be painful for you. You can also use more pressure with the knobble by applying your weight against the tool. Sometimes your masseuse cannot get the correct angle or applying pressure is difficult at particular angles and again this is where the knobble becomes the better tool.

The weighted tubular bar is most effective when working large muscle groups. It's highly effective when using it on the triangulares sterni, the pectorals, the gluts, the hamstrings and quadriceps, back muscles, and the muscles under the rib cage. Because it covers a greater area, it can simultaneously work 5 muscles at once. This tool does not work on areas like the neck, the top of the shoulders, the lats. These areas involve odd angles or locations where the bar is too big.

As your structure improves due to muscular changes and you reach road blocks where you are not sure what to work on, go back to the masseuse. Check for signs to see if it looks like your body is balanced and aligned. If you still need the chiropractor due to bones misaligning, then you are clearly not done yet and have more work ahead and that's where the masseuse can help you to get on track.

In my situation, when I thought I had done all I could on the neck, I was still needing the chiropractor and realized there was more work ahead. My hip needed a great deal of focus and once this had changed, it showed me that I wasn't done with the neck. As changes occur, alignments change, re-balancing makes adjustments and a neck that seemed great before the hip work, was no longer great after the hip work. So stay on track in using all of your tools and all of the signs because an unhappy muscle can appear happy if something is helping it out.

What You Experience with Muscular Changes

MUSCLES THAT ARE TRAPPED AND experiencing pressure begin to fight under the pressure. While in this pressure state it will feel like a hum that is electrically driven. I would describe it like electrical waves that restructure the knotted area. While the muscle is experiencing this it is important to keep the constant pressure until the muscle releases and the knot undoes itself. It is at this time you will feel the release and the muscle elongates and electrical waves stop. You may still have the knobble there or the masseuse there but there is no pressure as the muscle becomes pliable and relaxed and unbothered by the knobble. It is at this point you have success and can move on to the next locked up muscle.

It is important to remember that all muscles should be pliable and have give. If there is any tightness at all that is a problem that needs addressing. In fact, my problems were so extensive that my entire body had tightness and it appeared to me that it was on its way to becoming solid, which is very dangerous to one's health.

Most knotted or damaged muscles release within 90 minutes of constant pressure. The worst ones always take longer. As your healing is fully underway you will have muscles that will release within a couple of minutes. As always breathing deep breaths will make the process take less time. And it is at that moment when the release occurs that will finally have that big full breath that you had trouble achieving before.

If you experience a muscle that refuses to release and there are no signs of electrical waves within the muscle and you've given it 90 minutes, please stop. The muscle is tight because of another muscle and you will have to find the muscle that is the real culprit. For me this was very important with my back muscles. They just refuse to release because they are not the muscles to blame for the tightness. They were simply responding to the locked up muscles of my front. Once you have treated the muscles that caused the bad muscle in your back, you can then revisit it and get it to relax. But I found in most cases when you release the correct muscles on your front side, the muscles on your back side will relax automatically because your structure improved.

Be In Charge of Your Health

I KNOW IT'S PRETTY CUSTOMARY to go to your health professional to seek help when you suspect something isn't right and you should. The longer a problem exists, the worse it gets and affects your entire body. The problem lies in that we look to our health professional to solve our problem and sometimes they can't or won't. The health profession does what they can in a cost effective manner. And that's when your needs may not be met.

Let me describe my personal example. I had a broken clavicle (collar bone) from a car accident which would not heal in the customary way. I asked them to do surgery, they said no, saying they had to use all other methods possible. It wasn't until 10 months after the initial accident that they finally gave me the surgery that I knew was necessary and even then I had to fight for it. My doctor (head of their surgery department) said I should just live with it broken as it's not weight bearing to living normally. However, I wasn't living normally since I was a gymnast and in that case the collar bone was weight bearing for my hobby. I also thought it was inappropriate to have an arm that felt disconnected from the rest of me. I've literally never looked at the health profession the same again. How dare they only see their costs and weigh it against my ability to have my life back the way it was. Then there was the fact that this surgery required a bone graft from the hip.

I left the hospital with my steel plate in my collar bone and a left leg I had to drag around until it started working again. They then monitored my collar bone and later removed the plate and I healed. However, while trying to heal from a neck injury, I found that the hip with the bone graft had changed and was a factor in my neck healing; I literally had to heal the hip before I could heal the neck. Why didn't they ever think about the hip again once the graft was taken? Was their ignorance a major contributor to my neck injury? Was it that they didn't know they did damage? Why didn't they ever monitor the hip? I mean, they had moved muscles around to get the graft, yet no care was given in its recovery. They knew I was leaving the hospital and couldn't walk, surely that had some clue.

I want to believe they didn't know, but I also saw how their costs in my case were more than they wanted to spend. So how many people aren't getting what they need because of costs. How many things are just forgotten because they don't want to address them? We have to always keep in mind that hospitals are a business just like any other. They exist to make money.

Chiropractic is quite similar, their intentions appear good and I'm sure they feel they are doing a service. However the reality is only a few chiropractors offer massage and include it as part of their service. At least with massage they are showing an attempt to heal you the best way they know how. If they don't offer massage as part of their service, you should not use them because it is the muscles that cause the bones to misalign. So if the root cause is never improved by the chiropractic office, and they simply crack the bones to your correct alignment and the next day the muscles throw them back out again, you are simply at a point of just throwing your money at them. Again, they exist to make money and we have to always keep that in mind. Are they doing what's right for us? They will tell you that you need it, but what you need is to heal. Ask them how will you heal with what they alone are doing.

Finding the right masseuse is also important. Every masseuse has either different training or different experiences or different ways of handling their approach. Find a masscuse who is willing to listen to you and your needs. It's not enough that they are good at massage, they need to be good at listening as well. I have seen tons of masseuses who refuse to use their elbows and then spend the hour complaining that applying the pressure needed is hurting them. By using the elbows, then can elongate their career and give their thumbs a break. But the excuse you get is that they can't feel with their elbows and I understand that point of view, however, you do have 2 arms. Have them use one hand to trap and feel the muscle while the elbow does the heavy lifting (applying pressure). This way the masseuse will always be feeling what's happening and can feel secure about what he's doing. As the customer, keep your masseuse aware of any changes you are experiencing and try to stay calm and relaxed and focused on your breathing.

I think the biggest problem is that we want to trust the health professional, and in fact what we need to do is to get involved in the process. Ask them; what should I focus on doing, how can I help the process. Much of us doesn't ask and don't get. Those chiropractors and doctors get paid good money; let's make them work for it by asking the right questions and being a major player to improving our health. I have found that in asking these questions and they don't know the answers that it's time to find another health professional. If a chiropractor cannot tell you what muscles to work on to improve where he's adjusting, then that's a problem. In my experience that happens in a lot of chiropractic offices, and quite frankly it's a factor that needs to change. However if we never make them work for your answers, the industry won't change and won't improve.

So in conclusion, it's very important to get involved and leading the way to improving your health. I know it's our first instinct to be respectful of doctors, but they are not Gods. The body is a highly complex mechanism and it strikes me that because it is so complex means that no one can know everything about it. As individuals, we need to see our bodies as something we need to be constantly learning about. No one will have our self interest as strongly as ourselves. Be in charge.

Should You Get Chiropractic Care?

As you have determined your problems are muscular, should you seek chiropractic care? Chiropractic care should be used within reason. By all means do not go 3 times a week because it is waste of money. Once a week or once every 2 weeks is enough visits to the chiropractor. You will always feel better after your adjustment, almost euphoric. What this does is to help you see how you should be. The new alignment is usually temporary with muscular issues, so don't expect it to last long. However, use it as a gauge to judge as to how you are progressing in your healing. If your adjustment lasted longer than last time, you could be on the road to healing. If there's no change, and you always lose your adjustment by morning than you need to consider that you haven't found the problem yet. And sometimes finding the problem can take awhile. Be prepared to look for the problem in areas you didn't expect. For example, my neck was always out the next morning or even hours after the adjustment and I had given great care to the neck, so I had to look in other areas, and it was determined that I needed to fix my hip in order to fix the neck.

The most important factor you need to gain from your chiropractic experience is to see how the muscles adjust. In the first hour after the adjustment, things usually feel really good. It is in the second through fifth hours afterwards that you need to really pay attention. First off, don't plan on any physical endeavor after your adjustment. And lift nothing heavier than a gallon of milk. Plan for a calm relaxing time, where you have the chance to really feel what's happening. After your euphoric period, there is a period where the muscles have realized there's a change, and begin to feel strained. Not long after that, your muscles will make their own adjustments trying to compensate for those strained ones because they are weak or have knots and need attention. It's the strained ones that are your problem areas and usually show themselves for a brief period of time before giving up and allowing the body to make the changes it needs to relieve the pressure. That's why we really need to concentrate on feeling for them. And that is also why by the next morning or evening hours after the adjustment, you will feel those initial straining muscles earlier are better, however, in doing so, you have also lost your chiropractic adjustment. As usual, the muscles won out over the bones alignment. This is why the chiropractic is necessary. It gives you the clues you need to heal but only if you're paying attention.

How Important is Stretching?

STRETCHING ON ITS OWN CAN be healing. I had plantar fasciitis as one of my health issues and even though its root cause was my neck injury, my instinct was to heal it as its own injury. So I proceeded to see the doctor and get cortisone shots in each foot. The shots worked for about 2 weeks and then the pain was back. A friend of mine advised me not to get too many of those shots. So I asked about other methods and was told that it could be healed by stretching. Well, stretching is something I have always done and believed in so I dived right in. I worked my feet every day, putting them through the full range of motion even though it was painful to do. And in a matter of weeks, the pain was gone, my feet were better.

Not only can stretching cause healing, but it can also be looked at as a maintenance to keeping full range of motion. And one can spend some 5 minutes each day stretching and the reward will last all day.

Stretching can also bring awareness to a deficiency in movement. One day when I felt my neck injury recovery was about half way solved, I did neck stretches, leaning my head toward each shoulder and holding it and allowing the muscle to relax in the stretched position. I found that my range of motion was different from one side to the other. Where I could lean my head to the right shoulder some 60 degrees, I was only able to get 35 degrees out of the left side. This is another example of a sign I couldn't ignore. I still had a ways to go and even though continued stretching can help this issue, I needed to unlock some really damaged muscles in my neck in a more progressive nature.

The Egoscue Center recommends doing exercises and stretching as a healing method to correct the alignment problems they discover. And while I'm a huge advocate for stretching and exercises, there is some damage that needs a more progressive nature. The muscle itself needs to change. In that way, a knobble (massage tool) works the best to unlock the damage. Because it works on just one segment of the muscle that has a problem whereas stretching works to elongate the entire length of the muscle. But the whole muscle may not be a problem; it just may be a particular spot or maybe it's only at the attachments of the muscle. Sometimes you have to use the knobble near where the muscle inserts into the bone, or as close to the bone as our body will allow. Stretching cannot solve this issue either. But even though stretching cannot heal a particular spot, it can aid in the health of the muscle from developing new problem spots.

To Use Heat or Ice

CHRONIC MUSCULAR PAIN IS NOT an acute injury and therefore ice should not be used. Heat is appropriate, as it tries to relax tense or damaged or strained muscles. I try to remember to use heat as a precursor to playing tennis knowing that I'm still in the process of healing. It loosens them up before exerting them. And can be very affective after doing your physical activity to try to calm the muscles down after the exertion. Heat is also very good after a massage or other muscle work. It can also be used prior to massage because it can assist the masseuse in getting the muscle to change. It's best to have one of those heating pads that you pop in the microwave and 3 minutes later you have heat that will last like 15 minutes. I was in so much muscular pain at one point, that I took my heating pad to work every day and used it while working.

A funny story I have is, one day I had a tennis match in 95-100 degree weather which has never been good for me as I have a problem playing in extreme heat. I brought ice to my match and wrapped it in a wet towel and placed it on my shoulders and used it in the changeovers to prevent over-heating. It was working at first but being that most of my muscular damage was to the neck and shoulders, it back-fired big time. I found that 2/3 through the match my neck and shoulders seized up and I could no longer lift my arms up to do the serve. As it turned out, I still won the match but had to finish it with an underhand serve, obviously putting me at quite a disadvantage. Instead of winning 6-4, 6-4, it went on to a third set tie-break. So I realized that using ice on bad muscles is a big no-no. And if I really needed the ice I'd have to figure somewhere else to place it.

So please, do not use ice if your problems are muscular. And as for heat, I found no down side to using it as much as you want as long as the muscles do not become dependent on it.

What if I Have Scoliosis?

Scoliosis is the spine having curvatures where it should be straighter. Because of this lacking, the best thing to do is to make sure your musculature is strong to compensate. So in essence, a physical activity or sport is best. I personally have the S curve and my sister has a C curve and we both did gymnastics and we both were competitive. Don't tell yourself I can't do it because you have this slight handicap. And some people compete and no one can tell you have this handicap. Some people have a severe curvature and need surgery or a cast, but that's only the extreme and is not that common. I personally competed as a collegiate gymnast and did just fine with this slight handicap. I later did get chiropractic adjustments for other areas, and they usually adjusted my spine where the curve went from one side to my other side.

I'm not convinced the scoliosis was a factor in my caving inward process, especially because scoliosis is a bone issue and my problems were muscular. And my muscular problems were definitely a derivative of past injuries. Did the scoliosis weaken the bones and therefore more likely to lose their chiropractic adjustments, then maybe so, it's really hard to tell. It's best to be safe and look for signs more frequently if you have this slight handicap. It's really easy to blame everything, but the major culprit remains with the muscles and how they have reacted to injury over time.

Should I Workout While Trying to Make Muscular Changes?

I WOULD NOT WORK OUT with weights as in weightlifting because it is counter-productive to making muscular changes. You are literally trying to strengthen and built up an unbalanced body. At this point you are adding more bad muscle because you haven't resolved the muscle problems you currently have. I would work out with stretches for sure and even aerobic or cycling. I personally continued my tennis and it was pretty painful to do it that way, so I say it is up to you and your life style. And my healing process may have been shortened if I was able to skip the tennis. I worked out through all my changes and the one thing I can tell you is that pain from changes can direct you to know what to work on next. It's loud and clear what to work on when you are combining physical activity with muscle work. So I see it as you can find some advantage in whatever you decide.

Always give the body 24 hours after any major change before being physical. There were times in my healing process where the change was so extreme that I even waited 48 hours. The one thing I did almost every day though was to use my stationary bicycle for 15 minutes a day and I would always do the muscle work directly after the bike riding. Therefore your next riding is 24 hours later, but at least you got it in every day. Because the body really does need this 15 minutes a day as a daily ritual; it staves off weight gain and produces a healthy heart. I would call this 15 minutes a day a bare minimum to being healthy and lively.

So whether you decide to continue your sports or to just do your 15 minutes a day, either will work. Just don't do the weight lifting, it can only make matters worse when working towards muscular healing.

My Story

I GREW UP LIKE MOST kids, going to school and choosing hobbies. I discovered gymnastics when I was 13 and was incredibly excited about my new sport. I was strong but not very flexible so I had to work hard on what I lacked. I easily moved through the levels and joined the Hayward Area Recreation Dept. gymnastics team. I was doing well until I had some injuries. The first was a broken/dislocated elbow. I returned knowing my elbow may never be the same but I didn't let that stop me. Then my next injury was to my knees (hyper extending them, an ACL injury) and between the knees and the elbow my parents took me out of it permanently at the age of 16. So I began my return at 18 after leaving home by teaching gymnastics as a side job. It allowed me to dabble with the sport, not getting too serious. However, the drive was still there and my injuries were healing and I learned that if I was very careful with my landings (bent knees, feet together) that I could start to learn new skills and I decided to take gymnastics at Cal-State Hayward. The coach watched my progress during the class and at the end asked me to join her college team. I competed during the '82-'83 season and had lots of success learning new skills, but the nagging knee injury did return and I ended the season only competing on beam and bars. I absolutely loved this sport and continued to learn and work out for 27 years. But during that 27 years, I landed on my head 4 times. Like any gymnast does, you fall, get right back up and do the skill again. It happens every day, no big worry. I was so strong I never looked back. But years later, things like that, that go unaddressed, catch up to you.

I later had a car accident at the age of 33, where a guy had a seizer and partially hit the car in front of me and then proceeded to hit me head on. I had a broken clavicle (collar bone) and a couple broken ribs and a totaled vehicle. The clavicle refused to heal because I was still so very flexible by then. After 10 months, the doctors finally allowed me to have the surgery that would heal me in 2 years. And at the age of 35 I returned to gymnastics. For some reason, every time I had a set-back, it inspired me to return. Something about getting right back up there and doing it again was in-bread in me, even though before the accident I was feeling like I was ready to retire. But I never felt like I reached my best, it was still out there. So at age 35, I continued and even learned new skills, putting my aerial cartwheel and round-off flip-flop on the balance beam for example. Anyways, for my 40th birthday I retired and took up tennis. Yes, it's much safer, no more worrying about landing on one's head.

Tennis was a great transition as it allowed me to be extremely physical while still having to use my brain, only for strategy instead. There was no way I can change to a sport that didn't require brainwork.

At the age of 44, my neck injury started speaking to me. My right arm stopped working properly. I had pretty much just had a power game in tennis and with a right arm that turned into a noodle and could only do drop shots instead of drives, it was time to face that fact that my 4 falls on the head had finally caught up to me. My neck had also been very stiff, but now it was affecting the whole body. Soon after I sought medical care, I developed plantar fasciitis. And soon after that I had repeated hamstring injuries. I was a mess. I even had to buy shoes with side wholes because my feet were hot every time I played tennis. My medical care at the time, was getting monthly acupuncture treatments. Kaiser's catch phrase is that you have to say you have long-term chronic pain, and they'll send you to acupuncture. After the first year, my acupuncturist said it was time to start massage again, that his therapy couldn't do it alone. I had stopped getting massages for a period because everyone was saying they couldn't massage the bone in my neck. I told them it's not bone, it's damaged muscle. My acupuncturist had compared my neck to piano wire. I had to face it that no one wanted to work on my neck. But he said it was time to try the massage again, so I tried, and it was pretty futile, but there was a hint of the muscle being more receptive. At this point, it became a matter of finding the right masseuse. After 3 years of acupuncture, I was told they couldn't help me anymore, the acupuncture was not going to solve my problem. It was the most real thing anyone ever told me, someone who was finally honest. The acupuncturist told me that my problem was structural. I was like, what does that mean. It literally means that the body has taken on a new shape, one that can't heal, a shape that needs to change back to its original state in order for healing to begin. So he told me to go to this place called The Egoscue Center. So I contacted them, and my appointment consisted of measuring my alignment by taking a picture in front of a graph type wall, converting those pictures to a computer, and giving me measurements and degrees of what's off. I was flabbergasted. My head was tilted over, my head was turned to one side, I had a high hip, and a high shoulder and my feet weren't pointing equally and you could see more of one side of me then the other, and my left arm literally hung in front of me while the other hung on the side. It was as if my left side had completely collapsed in towards the right. So they analyzed my problems and came up with exercises. While I was learning the exercises I became aware that while lying on my back, I couldn't even get my shoulder blades to touch the floor evenly. Even lying on my back, the left shoulder couldn't touch the floor. They wanted me to make regular visits but I could not afford that and promised to return after completing the exercises and making progress. It was about this time I met the most fabulous masseuse. He understood how to release muscles. He came to my home and worked on my muscles every week. Finally, someone who's not afraid of working on the neck. Someone who understands that my damage is extensive and requires using his elbows instead of his hands. Someone who can pin one muscle down for 1 ½ hours and wait it out until the muscle finally caves. He did for me what no one in my life could do, and I've seen many therapists and many masseuses over the years. I saw chiropractors as well but never did any healing from them. This gentleman worked on my muscles for 2 years visiting me each week. He changed my life. He got me out of the pain I was in day in and day out. He was a life saver. But by now it's 2009 and I lost my job due to the economy and I can't afford my masseuse any more. I had to solve my injuries myself. Now I did return to Eqoscue before the job loss, and was hugely disappointed that my healing was only half way. I needed to come up with something on my own. But what? I had my muscle tool, a knobble, and would try to use it and place it where I had the latest discomfort. Using my rocking chair lying across it sideways and wedging my shoulder in the seat-bed and my neck against the arm of the chair, I was able to work my neck by placing the knobble in my neck with the backside against the chair. I made huge progress with my neck doing this but I still wasn't changing the body enough. The neck felt better but the body didn't. What was going on? I would play tennis and kept feeling like no matter what I did to the neck, my left shoulder would pull forward. So one day I thought, lift up one side of the rocking chair and place the runner on my front while lying on my back and aim the runner to the left side. I could feel muscular changes and when I got up I felt better. God bless that rocking chair. No seriously, I realized that I had to find something else that could effectively have enough weight and could be aimed at specific areas of my front and not be so cumbersome as a full chair or have the runner actually do damage. OK so I found something almost as ridiculous, but it worked. My stationary exercise bicycle had tubular bases. I would place one base on my chest (specifically to open the left side). They were heavy so the weight caused almost instant changes to muscle and they were large enough to release some 5 muscles at once. All I had to focus on was my breathing, long deep breaths. And I was vaguely aware that it was the exhale that produced the most change, when the air is out and you need to breath again. There was an amazing amount of bad muscle just to the left of the sternum with the base placed horizontally. Diagonally I placed the base across the left ribs (never along the line of the rib) and again, more huge changes. I got releases this way from my clavicle to sternum connection and even hip changes. The results were staggering. I would play tennis and I felt years younger and had a whole new body. I was immediately aware that more parts where working and I better learn to control all that was now functional. I felt like that 12 year old girl again who was always tripping on my way to school, of course until I started gymnastics and went from being a klutz to a swan. What strikes me the most is that if I had continued with the massage it would have taken so much longer to heal as this way more muscles could heal all at once. It was so instant. And the feeling is amazing. And you feel so alive. However, you have to understand that change is painful. The body seems to produce ripple effects throughout. When you do have a major change, it typically feels great and you do a physical activity and you'll get a lot of soreness. That's the muscles adapting to the new alignment. And because of this, you always want to wait 48 hours before doing more muscle work. This applies to the weighted bar as well. The body has to accept the changes before you can make corrections, because the body finds ways of adapting, however the body might not chose the way you had intended it to go. So you will need to repeat the weighted bar until the body finally accepts the alignment you want from it. So for every 2 steps forward, you get one step back effect. And your body literally wants to heal the muscles in a reverse order of how they became damaged. It has taken me 5 ½ years to heal from the time I began at the acupuncturist. And even though the acupuncturist couldn't heal me, I know that his work on my neck was instrumental in allowing the muscles to change as so many have tried to work them for so long. And I have to tell you, I just might go dabble with some gymnastics, even though I just turned 50. Sometimes, it's your own ingenuity that can save the day. Never give up. Healing is possible. I am proof, I suffered in pain for 20 years and now I'm pain-free. Now I'm ready to go to back to The Egoscue Center because I want to hear that my alignment is the way it's supposed to be and my structure has been corrected.

www.ingramcontent.com/pod-product-compliance
Lightning Source LLC
Chambersburg PA
CBHW050335290526
45785CB00006B/2509